WELLNESS POWER
A CONSUMER rEVOLUTION

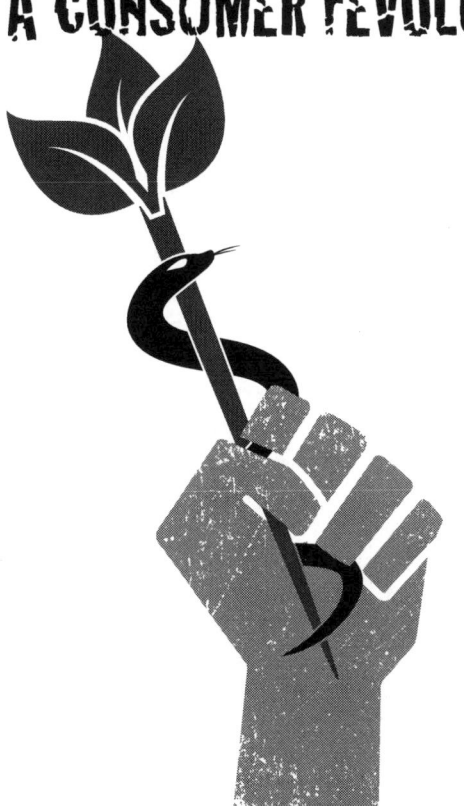

SUSAN FREDERICK

Wellness Power

Copyright © 2018 Susan Frederick

All rights reserved. No part of this book may be reproduced or transmitted in any form or by any means without written permission of the author.

ISBN 978-1-7208-5996-3

*This book is dedicated to those we love
who left us far too soon…and to those
who suffered needlessly because we did
not yet understand the secrets of wellness.*

Here's to the Revolution!

Salud!!

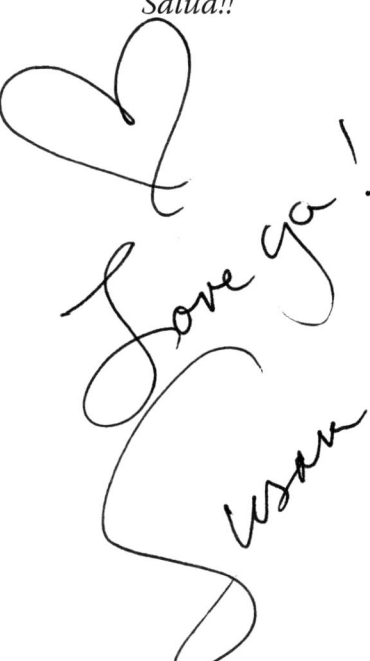

Table of Contents

Preface 1
Introduction 3
1 Enough of Sick and Tired. 5
2 Two Golden Rules 13
3 Deficiencies Cause Trouble 21
4 They Didn't Know What They Didn't Know. . 29
5 A Consumer Revolution. 39
6 Finding the Truth in a Marketing Maze 47
7 Creating the Habit. 57
8 Affording Wellness 67
9 Sharing the Gift. 75
10 Stress Free for Real 89
11 It's Your Call. 101
Epilogue. 109
Suggested Reading. 111

Preface

Three years ago I changed the course of my life.

You can too.

It's worth it.

And it's time.

Introduction

Before he was my husband, Don Frederick was my best friend. He moved in across the street when I was 13 and we were together almost every day thereafter. When he finished graduate school, we got married and had a son. Five years later, he was jogging around the high school track with some buddies when he suddenly felt dizzy. He stopped to get his balance. His buddies thought he fainted. But he didn't. He was dead.

It was three years ago my mom was diagnosed with Parkinson's disease. She'd had essential tremors in her hands for years, but they didn't call it Parkinson's—until then.

Both my grandfathers died of heart attacks. One of them I never had a chance to know. He died when my dad was 17.

My father had bypass surgery when he was younger than I am now. It worked for awhile. But we've been without him now 18 years.

A year ago my best friend's sister died of colon cancer. She was 52.

One of my younger friends has Lupus. She's almost 30 and just had a baby.

A business friend struggled with fibromyalgia for 12 long years. Some days the pain was so intense she could hardly move. The doctors said it would get worse as she got older. She was 42.

When my daughter was a teenager she babysat a little girl named Jill. Three years ago Jill died of Leukemia. She was 17.

I could go on, but you get the drift. And you could make your own list, I'm sure.

Here's my question:

How much of this are we going to take before we holler "Uncle?"

Chapter One

Enough of Sick and Tired

Yes, and how many deaths will it take till we know that too many people have died?
—Bob Dylan

One

As a personal and business coach, I talk with people from California to Florida who are vibrant, energetic entrepreneurs. They're innovative, enthusiastic, committed to their dreams. Many of them wrestle with health issues that don't seem to have solutions.

In case you haven't noticed, this country has a health problem. Big. Huge. I could quote statistics, but I doubt if I need to. You know what I'm talking about. You also know what they've told us. From hot flashes to arthritis, they've told us it's just part of getting older. They've told us no one understands the cause of auto-immune diseases, or allergies, or cancer. They have treatments, of course. Drugs. Some of them have helped relieve our symptoms. Some of them haven't. Some of them have had side effects worse than the original problem. And no matter how you slice it, they haven't touched the underlying problem. They weren't expected to.

I have a confession to make. This is not an issue I cared much about. Mostly I walked around it, stepped over it. Like anything else you see too often, you get to where you don't really see it at all. You take it for granted. That was me. I didn't think about it. People were sick. People were tired. People died. That was life as I knew it. I accepted whatever medical theories and explanations (or lack of them) there were. And I assumed that getting older meant winding up with body problems—and sometimes, even when you're not older, your body just goes haywire for no reason. I mean, what can you do?

Exactly. What can you do?

Three years ago something inside me started to wake up. The looming shadow I hadn't been willing or able to see became visible, and menacing—like a giant specter silently threatening to overtake us.

Enough of Sick and Tired

At the same time the realization dawned on my endarkened brain that it simply was not supposed to be this way. Not only was it not supposed to be this way—it didn't have to be this way.

It was a revelation that changed my life. And I can't take any credit for discovering it. Someone brought it to me. Just like someone who handed you this book is bringing it to you.

I'll give myself this much credit, though. I pursued it. Well, okay, not right at first. I admit to being gently pestered by someone who was willing to risk annoying me. And I resisted for awhile. I mean—who has time to devote to such things? I was a single parent with a million commitments, none of which included checking out new information. But eventually, thank God, I gave up and listened.

I listened to doctors who had information that a lot of other doctors hadn't yet encountered. I watched live and recorded lectures by researchers who had seen health conditions we thought to be irreversible, nevertheless reverse themselves. Over the last three years I've read books, research papers, and peer reviewed medical studies. And I've listened to hundreds of people with personal experience tell what has happened to them. Anecdotal, they call it. But when you put all the scientific and experiential puzzle pieces together, the picture it forms is extremely exciting. Quite frankly, it's a picture that could change the quality of life for pretty much everyone on this planet.

However (and this is a BIG however), there's something that's been with us since before Galileo upset the pope with the news that the sun didn't revolve around the earth, after all. Whenever a new awareness brings to light things that threaten to alter a previous perspective, there are only three options available:

1. Deny, doubt or ignore (do not take time to research) the emerging facts and just keep rolling with your old beliefs.

2. Acknowledge the emerging facts, but don't make any personal changes because _____ (fill in the blank with whatever suits you.)

3. Research the facts, give your cobwebby head a shake, then get up on your hind legs and take responsibility for your own future.

As we all know, the pope picked number one, which makes him look really dumb to us today and kept the world in the dark ages for I don't know how many more years. Ultimately, of course, the truth got out. It usually does.

But here's the deal. When it comes to our health, we don't have to wait until the pope gives us the okay to get out of our own personal dark ages. I'm telling you—there's some new light out there. We just have to be willing to let it in.

Chapter Two

Two Golden Rules

When accurate information can't get through the too-thick wall of profit—we're the ones who lose.

Two

When I first began to study this information, I was skeptical. If even half of what I was finding out was true, surely it would have been headline news in every newspaper in the world. I guess that shows my intractable naiveté. I seem to keep forgetting the golden rule. Not the one that Jesus advocated. The other one:

Them that has the gold makes the rules.

Even in this burgeoning and unstoppable information age, the mainstream media is still owned by the mega corporations. They're the ones who buy multi-million dollar television ads and have lobbyists for every legislator in Congress. Basically, their money tells the media what to say and the government what to do. Is it true that money talks? You better believe it. And big money talks BIG.

In the medical arena, it's the pharmaceutical corporations that own America. Medical schools depend on their donations and the FDA depends on their research. Medical doctors are educated, fed, and catered to by pharmaceutical reps around the country. Even the yearly CME (Continuing Medical Education) classes that doctors are required to take in order to keep their licenses, are financed primarily by pharmaceutical companies.

So what happens when new information enters the scientific community that could transform the medical landscape without benefiting the pharmaceutical industry?

Not much. With doctors as busy as they are, they hardly have time for their own families, much less for extra curricular research. And as insulated as they are by big pharma, non-pharmaceutical information rarely filters through that membrane.

That's why your doctor may not know about this. Hey, it's not his fault. He's a product of the system. We all are. That's the problem.

What about the Internet? Thank God corporate America doesn't own that...yet.

True enough. But if you've been on the net lately you know it's a hodge-podge of pretty much everything. From marketing to matchmaking to things we hope our kids will never see or hear—the Internet is like a huge wall of multi-faceted graffiti. Anyone can post anything. It's free speech at its best and worst. The obvious dilemma is that you don't know if anything you see is true. You don't even know who's actually posting it—or why.

Just recently, a web researcher in the health arena called into question certain "quack-buster" type websites for fraudulent posts designed to discourage trade with their competitors. The authorities are now pursuing it and hopefully, they'll shut it down. But the reality is that negative Internet advertising is powerful. Corporations can shoot bullets at their emerging competition by covertly paying an "objective third party" to post faux research that makes the other company look bad. Internet savvy consumers know that and take it with a grain of salt. But less savvy consumers assume the posts are valid. There's no telling how much defamation and lost business honest companies have suffered because of an "objective third party," which turns out to be none other than their integrity deficient competitors.

On top of that the golden boys use lawsuit leverage. Companies with deep pockets can easily afford to sue smaller companies whose success may threaten their dominance. Did you happen to see the cover of Forbes magazine toward the end of 2006? It highlighted a law firm that actually recruited class action plaintiffs (they paid two of them over a million dollars!) so they could sue up-and-coming companies with enough cash to make for a nice settlement but not enough money to fight back. The article reported billions of dollars had been bilked over the last few years from companies whose insurers opted to settle rather than face the predictable avalanche of legal and court costs. Thankfully, every attorney in that sleazy law firm is now under federal indictment.

It's too bad about the smudged reputations and lost profits of the victims.

Oops. Sorry.

All that to say that, in the short term, at least, "them that has the gold makes the rules." But only until. There's always an until. Because in the end, the second golden rule can't trump the first. Eventually, someone somewhere stands up and calls it what it is. Then someone else recognizes the truth of it and sings along. And another and another until it becomes a whole chorus, and then a grass roots movement. Call it evolution or revolution, it's the kind of thing that got this country started in the first place and it's the force that will ultimately triumph. It's called the truth. It's why Galileo is the history book hero instead of the pope who tried to shut him up. That's the great thing about the truth. Once it's actually out there, even "them that has the gold" can't oppose it and win.

Nope. Not even if they're the pope.

Chapter Three

Deficiencies Cause Trouble

*Without proper structure and function
at a cellular level, optimal health is
simply not a possibility.
In other words,
You gotta have your littlest parts in place
—or something bad is going down.*

Three

Here's a wild idea for you: God made the human body to self-repair. Actually, that's not a controversial idea (except for the God part, which some dispute.) Case in point: Knick yourself with a razor and watch what happens. It bleeds. You put a pinch of Kleenex on it and it stops. Now, check it in a day or two. Poof, the knick is gone.

Nobody argues that the body isn't meant to heal. Of course it is. That's what it does for a living. Those who know these things tell us that everyone gets mini-versions of cancer (mutant cells whose DNA has somehow gotten screwed up) all the time. It's normal. The immune system is in constant surveillance, however, and as soon as it detects said cells, it triggers a process that gets rid of them. No problem.

If you get a bacterial infection of some kind, the body knows just how to deal with it. It sends anti-bodies to attack the invader and defend the homeland. When the deed is done, it calls off the troops and sends them back home. No problem.

You need to understand something. In the physical world, your body is your own best friend. It will never betray you. It will always do its very best to keep you going, to protect and defend you against anything that would do you harm. Even when you ignore it, mistreat it, expose it to toxins, viruses, bacteria, stress—the body has its own recovery programs to put you back in the driver's seat, unless (there's that unless again) it is deficient in something.

Deficiencies are a big problem. That's not controversial. Try fighting a war without enough body armor and see what happens. Try building a car without all of its parts. Try growing a plant without enough water or sunlight. It can't be done. And human bodies that don't have what they need to fulfill on their commission will not be able to take care of you. It's that simple.

You may have read the story of Captain Cook and the thousands of British sailors that got scurvy on the lengthy voyages across the ocean. First, their gums started bleeding. What they didn't realize was that everything inside was bleeding too because their connective tissue was eroding. Thousands of them died. No one understood why. The doctors tried to figure it out. They tried everything they knew to help. Nothing did.

Finally, Captain Cook hired a botanist to travel with them and experiment with different "cures." The upshot of it was that the men with scurvy who were fed citrus fruits (oranges and limes) recovered. And those who ate the citrus fruits all along never got it at all. The doctors of that time scoffed at the botanist's conclusions, but in the end, he was correct. Citrus fruit prevented scurvy. Years later they discovered why. Scurvy turned out to be a vitamin C deficiency.

When my son, Matt, was a teenager he loved basketball and hated vegetables. He mainly liked canned ravioli, pizza, and hamburgers with nothing but meat, bread and ketchup. I was a single mom who didn't like to hassle her kids about food. So I didn't.

One day he came to me complaining about a patch on his leg where the hair wouldn't grow. "It looks weird," he told me. "What's wrong with it? It looks like goose flesh. I want you to take me to the dermatologist."

But dermatologists cost money. I didn't have any. That was a problem. Coincidentally (or synchronistically, if you believe in that), about that time I ran across a recording by a nutritionist discussing the symptoms of vitamin deficiencies. One of them was vitamin A, which is derived primarily from green and yellow vegetables. You'll never guess what one of the symptoms was. Goose flesh where hair won't grow. Bingo. I bought some Vitamin A and fed him the amount the nutritionist recommended for the amount of time she recommended. Result? Normal leg with hair and a happy boy.

Deficiencies Cause Trouble

That's a small thing, I know. You can survive without leg hair (albeit not happily if you're a 16 year old boy who plays basketball.) But other deficiencies have heavier consequences. Scurvy can kill you. Rickets can cripple you. Calcium deficiencies can leave you with bones that are porous like sponges and snap like a twig. And there are other deficiencies that are just as serious. One of them we have only recently discovered.

Chapter Four

They Didn't Know What They Didn't Know

*What most of us know:
Table sugar is not a health food.
What most of us don't know:
Scientists have discovered 8 sugars
that are absolutely crucial to health.*

Four

If you're old enough, you might remember back in the late 70's and 80's when potions made of aloe vera were all the craze. Drug stores sported gels and lotions and creams and drinks—all of them touting the magical properties of aloe vera—everything from healing teenage zits to disappearing age spots.

If you had a grandmother like mine, you might even recall an aloe vera plant sitting in the kitchen window—just in case you got a grease burn while you were frying eggs, or chicken for Sunday dinner. Someone told me once that aloe vera is mentioned five times in the Bible. I've never actually looked it up. But that's what I'm told.

So, what's the big deal about aloe vera, anyway? That's exactly what the FDA wanted to know back then. With all the marketing hype whirling around it, what was the actual truth? Did any of these aloe vera products have efficacy—or was it all just a big, catch-the-wave marketing trend taking gullible consumers for a ride? Basically, the FDA threw down the gauntlet and told the aloe vera potion makers to put up or shut up. Prove it works or else take it off the shelves. It was a big upset to the whole industry. Millions of dollars were at stake.

One company decided to defend their position by hiring a researcher to find the active ingredient in aloe vera and prove its efficacy. That research pharmacologist was a man named Bill McAnalley. What he found out (after years of tedious deductive experimental research) was surprising. He thought surely the active ingredient would be something dignified, like a protein or an amino acid. But no. The active ingredient in aloe vera turned out to be a long chain carbohydrate—a sugar molecule—called mannose. And it was a "labile" molecule, which meant it was vulnerable to heat and lost its efficacy within a couple of days. Oops. So much for all the aloe vera potions. Turns out they were mostly water.

But McAnalley wasn't done with his experimenting. Having found the active molecule, he determined to find a way to stabilize it. He did that and patented the process. So the company he worked with was able to market a stabilized aloe vera product that produced some amazing anecdotal results.

Long story short—mannose was discovered to be one of a group of 8 biologically active sugars (not to be confused with table sugar) that comprise a crucial communication network throughout the body. The electron microscope has now revealed that the surface of every one of your multi-trillion cells is covered with them in different configurations. Those configurations determine very important things—your blood type, for example. They also serve as docking stations for nutrients and hormones. And they convey messages. The messages they convey are critical to correct bodily functioning—and especially crucial to the immune system, which is responsible for recognizing internal dangers and mounting a defense.

It is also responsible for shutting it off when the job is done.

Let me be more specific. If the immune system doesn't get the message that a cell is mutant and should be eliminated, it won't eliminate it. Cancers can exist and multiply in a body for years before they are medically detectable. Early detection is the job of the immune system. So failure to detect and destroy is an immune system dysfunction.

Likewise, once the immune system destroys an invader, repressor cells should communicate a shutdown of the attack. If the communication is not delivered or received properly, the attack does not shut down. Healthy tissue is continuously attacked and inflamed for no apparent reason. This is called an auto-immune condition. There are currently over 80 diagnosed auto-immune conditions. Their names differ depending on what tissue is being attacked. But the dynamic is the same.

Since the 8 sugar molecules are pivotal in this communication network, it is logical to assume that if any of them are missing, the crucial messages might not be getting through. If you've ever tried dialing a phone number with a digit that was wrong, or emailing someone with a single letter out of place, you know what I mean. No matter how many times you try, you won't get through.

These 8 sugars are so crucial to your physical survival, that if you don't eat them, your body has to make them, which involves extensive enzymatic conversions and diverts a lot of energy you could use otherwise. But that wasn't necessary (except in emergencies) for hundreds of years because our ancestors did eat them. Tree saps, gums, seaweed, various fungi (don't wrinkle up your nose at me, those mushrooms you had on your steak last night are fungi) were on the daily menu. Fruits and roots, plants and leaves were picked and eaten the same day. No green harvesting of items not-yet-ripe, transported in railcars to grocery store shelves hundreds of miles away and eaten 3 weeks later when the necessary molecules are no longer there.

In today's world, green harvesting is the name of the game. Unless you're eating plants, fungi and tree sap that you're growing in your backyard, chances are you're one of the millions eating the standard

American diet. And of the 8 sugar molecules required for your cells to communicate, that diet includes 2. The other six are virtually non-existent.

It's a deficiency of major proportions—in an arena no one knew existed.

Along with his fellow researchers, Bill McAnalley began to grasp the implications of what he had discovered. Together, they began to put the aloe vera molecule (now called "acemannan") through its paces. They tested it in labs and on animals. They did clinical studies. And they began to predict the positive results with more and more accuracy. Eventually, they knew for sure that what they had could dramatically improve the health of the world. It was time to make a pharmaceutical out of this. It was time for FDA trials.

Alas, the first two trials failed to demonstrate drug-worthy characteristics. Lethal Dose (LD-50) is a test to establish toxicity levels. If you can kill 50% of the lab rats you can extrapolate the danger line for human subjects. But if your substance won't kill any rats at all—that's a problem. Second test was for drug interaction. Nope. Nada. Nothing.

Obviously, this subject had failed its drug interview. It was non-toxic at any level. It didn't interact with other drugs. By FDA standards it was a harmless food.

And the FDA doesn't deal with harmless foods. It deals with drugs and foods that are potentially harmful—like spinach with E-Coli in it. But a food that won't even kill a rat is not a candidate for FDA surveillance or approval.

It must have been a hard day for McAnalley and company. They thought they had a new drug that would change the world and it turned out to be something else. Little did they know the magnitude of what was about to happen next. Like all the rest of us, they didn't know what they didn't know.

Looking back with what we know now, it's obvious that the failure of drug trials was the best thing that could possibly have happened. The dismal failure was the gateway to a whole new world. What Bill McAnalley had discovered would never be a drug. It was indeed a food—a food that contained a class of nutrients never before recognized or understood. Like Christopher Columbus, he had started out to find a new route to the West Indies, and in the process he had accidentally run into America.

Chapter Five

A Consumer Revolution

Timing is everything…and now is the time.

Five

In the market place, as in the world at large, nothing new takes hold until people are ready. Timing is everything. That's why every revolution is preceded by a period of gradual evolution. Revolutions are simply Evolutions that have caught fire.

History is littered with innovations introduced before their time that didn't get a foothold. You don't know much about them because they didn't make it into the high school history books. What shows up there is what happened when people were ready.

Consider this. The American Revolution couldn't have occurred a minute before it did. In fact, it came very close to not occurring at all. There were plenty of colonial loyalists who felt that taking on the strongest military power in the world just might not be the best idea.

But over the years, more and more Americans had evolved past the point where they were willing to be intimidated by King George's England. They were second and third generation Americans whose English loyalty was mainly relegated to the family scrapbook. What they valued was their independence. And they valued it more than the passive peace of business as usual. In short, they were tired of kowtowing. It took time, but at some point the revolutionaries gained a hearing, then a foothold, and finally a revolution burst into flame that resulted in their freedom.

Evolution becomes Revolution. Only when the people are ready.

Bill McAnalley had run into something that could change the health of the world. And it wasn't a drug. It was a food—a food that contained critical components for human well-being. Magic bullets that caused cells to communicate with one another

A Consumer Revolution

and without which immune systems went into fail-safe mode, like hospitals that rely on generators when the power goes out. No discovery in 100 years had been this important to human health.

But how do you get something this valuable into the people's hands? Pharmaceutical companies dominated the medical landscape. They regulated the inroads to doctors and patients. Laws had even been passed to keep consumers from getting health related information from anyone outside that professional fold. So, how was anyone going to find out about this?

Small pockets of people around the country had shown an interest in vitamins and were buying things at health food stores. So, experimentally, the new product wound up there for a couple of years. Sitting there quietly on health food store shelves, it was probably the loneliest item of all. No one wanted it because no one knew what it was. If it wasn't a vitamin or a mineral—what was it? Labels don't say much. They aren't allowed.

The truth was—it wasn't time. And people weren't ready.

But things changed.

In 1994 the legislature passed a new law: The Dietary Supplement Health & Education Act, DSHEA. This remarkable piece of legislation dismantled the electric fence that had prevented the dispensing of health related information by anyone outside the medical profession. Legislators could see that the vitamin market was growing rapidly. Somehow on their own, people were learning that physical issues could be addressed with non-pharmaceuticals and that nutrition was a basic component of health. It had even come to light that missing nutrients could be a source of physical malfunctions. Clearly, nutrition impacted health. It was scientifically indisputable.

Nutrition. Imagine that. Medical doctors shook their heads. Some laughed. Others made jokes about expensive urine. Medical schools didn't have much input on nutrition. Most still don't. But it didn't matter. People were evolving. They began to wonder if there was more to health than waiting to be sick; something else to do besides sitting in a doctor's office and taking medicine when things went south.

A Consumer Revolution

They were tired of sick. They wanted to be well. And if there was a way to stay well they were willing to listen to new information with an open mind. It was the old "Galileo versus the pope" story all over again. And the people wanted to hear what Galileo had to say.

They were increasingly wary of the hazards of addressing every issue with another prescription. Nightly news told of some who had died from combinations of prescription drugs that had never been tested together. And, sometimes, they knew from personal experience, you didn't die. You just discovered that the side effects were worse than the problem. Surely, there were other options.

People were looking for new answers. But how ready were they? Were they ready to learn something they didn't know—something even their doctors might not know? Were they ready to take that much responsibility? McAnalley knew that's exactly what it would take if they were to experience the results he had seen in his research. He also knew that results would be all it took to set the thing on fire. Results. That's what they wanted. Results would be the spark that lit up the midnight sky and turned the emerging evolution into a raging revolution. A Wellness Revolution.

Chapter Six

Finding the Truth in a Marketing Maze

*When you're looking for a needle in a haystack,
It's helpful to have a magnet.*

Six

I know a guy named Ray who has diabetes. Not long ago I heard him mention some years ago a friend of his (named Sam) gave him a pile of written information about a natural product that some researcher (who happened to be seated next to him on an airplane) had told him about. The researcher guy had said there was some evidence it helped regulate hormone balance. And since insulin is a hormone, well, you can take it from there.

Since Ray was not only a multi-millionaire, but considered himself to be fairly intelligent, he was just a little insulted that Sam would think there was anything with any value out there that he wouldn't know about. Besides that, his doctor had been a friend since high school or college, so if there was anything out there that could help Ray keep his legs (he was on the list for amputation), his doctor most certainly would have told him. So why (said Ray to Sam) should he dig through a pile of documents about some Mexican Yam root?

So Ray was cantankerous and refused to look at the information. Sam insisted. Ray refused. Sam insisted. Finally, Ray gave in and read the pile of stuff. What he saw there shocked him. He took it to his doctor friend and asked him if he'd heard of it. Dioscorea Villosa was the proper name. Mexican Yam for short. To his amazement, the doctor had heard of it. He'd even read that it was a natural substance that could be of serious help to diabetics.

Ray was astounded and then angry. "Why didn't you tell me about it? Were you just going to cut off my legs without mentioning there might be something else that could help me?"

The doctor was apologetic, but explained that he couldn't recommend anything that was not "standard of care." When Ray asked why, he further explained that if Ray should sue him for any reason, having ever recommended something that wasn't "standard of care" could leave him professionally vulnerable. He could lose his license.

Long story short, Ray took the Mexican Yam stuff. And he still has his legs. He's the only male in his family to see his 60th birthday—and with legs still attached, no less. In his family, that's considered remarkable.

What's the moral of that story? It's not about yams and legs. And it's not about diabetes. It's about doctors. What you need to understand is where your doctor's coming from. I don't care if your doctor's been your best friend since the second grade, he (or she) still wants to keep his (or her) medical license. So he's (enough of the gender thing) not going to recommend anything that pharmaceutical companies and the AMA don't accept as "standard of care." The cutting, burning, and poisoning of cancer has been "standard of care" since the 1950's, for example. They may change the chemicals they use, but the process is the same. No matter that recovery is unpredictable and the side effects almost as hazardous as the disease itself. Hey, it's standard of care. In other words, medical tradition. And everyone knows it takes a long time for traditions to change.

Medicine is a serious sub-culture with its own rules of engagement. Step out of bounds, and if you get sued, you're dead in the water. So, don't expect your doctor to give his blessing to anything that doesn't lie within that circumference. I promise you it doesn't matter if it's totally harmless and couldn't kill a rat. If it comes in a bottle or a jar, it's suspect. And if he isn't educated on it, he won't recommend it. Even if he is, (given that there are accredited CME classes on the subject) he may still decline. Certain doctors I know are committed to specific nutritional supplements and use them personally and in their own families. Still, they will not mention them to patients. That's how paranoid they are about stepping over that "standard of care" boundary.

Another thing doctors know is that the dietary supplement industry is like the wild, Wild West before the sheriff came to town. It's basically an unregulated industry—and it will be that way until GMP's (good manufacturing practices) which are now legally required are finally enforced. Meanwhile, what that means to us consumers is that whatever we read on the labels of nutritional supplements may or may not actually be in the jar. It might be in some of the capsules, but not in others.

I know a research company that was running tests with combinations of anti-oxidants to measure their potential synergy. They ordered some green tea from a respected provider, but when they put it through its paces, they were puzzled to find it tested out at zero. It showed no ORAC value whatsoever. (Oxygen Radical Absorption Capacity is what ORAC stands for and is the way you measure anti-oxidant effectiveness.)

When they contacted the provider company, they asked why the product they tested would show no value. "Oh, we didn't know you were testing it. We thought you were in production."

"Why would you send a product with no value to be used for production?" they asked.

"Because that's what most companies use. They don't want the good stuff. It's too expensive."

Unfortunately, that's how it often works in an unregulated industry. Price trumps value. Quality and effectiveness are secondary considerations—if they're considered at all.

So, how do you know what's really good and what's just good marketing?

Excellent question.

Fortunately, there are ways to tell.

First off, insist on GMP's. Even though GMP's were not required by law until 2007, the best companies have already been implementing them for years. The others have obviously resisted regulation since they don't meet those standards. The new law requiring GMP's has given companies a fairly sizeable time window to get up to speed. So many of them still are not. Whatever you do, you definitely want to make sure the company you're dealing with has GMP's in place already.

Second, make sure they come from botanical sources and do not include genetically modified ingredients. Do not be fooled by the word "natural" that may appear on the label. A rock is "natural."

Petroleum is "natural." In this arena, the word "natural" tells you pretty much nothing.

Third, learn the science behind it. You don't need to be a scholar, but it's important to know what a product actually does and why it works. If it provides the raw material your endocrine system needs to make hormones—you should know that. And there should be scientific documentation to that effect. If it lends electrons to those roving free radicals that damage your cells and cause oxidative stress, and thus renders them harmless, you should know that. If it glycosylates your cells and facilitates message transfer that is so critical to your immune system—you should definitely know that.

Why is understanding so important? Two HUGE reasons:

One, you won't be seduced into buying dozens of supplements you don't really need just because you read about them in Prevention Magazine.

And two, you'll know exactly what role each product is playing in your body and how absolutely vital it is, so you won't quit or forget.

Forgetting and quitting have been the unfortunate death knell of many like yourself who started out with great intentions, but didn't really understand the cruciality of what they were doing. Inspiration without education has a short shelf life.

It doesn't really matter how good the products are that sit on your cabinet—if you forget or if you quit, you're going to lose the game. Hit or miss won't get the job done. Your body needs specific nutrients to keep itself in good repair—and it needs them every single day. Without consistency, optimum health will always stay just out of reach.

Inspiration and education will put you on the road, but only one thing will get you where you really want to go: Habit.

Chapter Seven

Creating the Habit

A new field called Nutrigenomics has shown that nutrients have been found to "turn on" beneficial genes and "turn off" harmful ones. In short, our diet and habits trump our genetics.

Seven

Habit: A pattern of activity that becomes virtually automatic through continuous repetition.

Is there anything I can say about habits that Mom and Dad, and Grandma and Grandpa, and Tony Robbins haven't already told us? Nevertheless, it bears repeating. Our habits are either our best friends or our worst enemies. While we're paying attention to other things, they're taking us quietly down the road to health and prosperity or else – the other way.

Let's face it. No one sets out to be unhealthy or overweight. It seems to happen all by itself. What we wanted was to be fit and trim—with a perfect blood pressure and cholesterol reading. But what we want is not the determining factor, is it? It's what we do. And what we do, ninety per cent of the time, is controlled by sheer habit.

You know that dish of ice cream you have every night after supper…those Hershey's kisses you love to pop in your mouth whenever you pass the candy jar…that little bit of extra dressing you put on your salad on top of those crunchy croutons? Those little bitty habits will walk you right down the primrose path to defeat without even a warning about the final destination.

Most of our habits aren't very significant in themselves. That's why it's so easy to believe they don't really matter. We're going to change them tomorrow anyhow, right? But oops, tomorrow didn't come. It's still today. And a habit that wins today, wins. Period. The great thing (and the worst) about a habit is that its effects are not immediate. They're cumulative. Sort of like the interest on your IRA (you do have one of those, don't you?) the results add up over time. And therein lies the benefit—or the rub.

Creating the Habit

In the health arena, habits will quite simply make you or break you.

And the crazy thing is you don't really have to do a lot to be healthy. You just have to do a few things consistently to keep the old body machine well oiled and in good repair for at least a hundred years.

1. Drink filtered water. (If you review an actual printout of what's in your local tap water, you will understand this rule and never dream of breaking it.)
2. Don't just sit there. (Give yourself at least 30 minutes of energetic activity daily.)
3. Breathe in till your stomach pooches out. (Several times a day fill up the lower part of your lungs as well as the top part.)
4. Make sure you get enough nutrition. (And that includes quality supplements since commercial farming, green harvesting, and chemical processing have pretty much stripped our food of everything except calories.)
5. Sleep at least 7 – 9 hours a night. (That's when your body does most of its repairs.)

6. Laugh a lot and have fun with the people you love.
7. Enjoy a relationship with God.

This last one should probably be the first one, but since some folks consider it controversial I figured I'd put it at the end. Feel free to leave it off the list if you want to. But just between us, personal experience suggests it's best to put it at the top, right before filtered water.

Seven habits. (Hey, wasn't there a best selling book by that title a few years ago? Maybe we're onto something here.)

None of them are difficult. And each of them has cumulative effects. In fact, they're synergistic. That means when you get several of them going at the same time, you get much more than a cumulative effect. (Instead of 2+2+2+2, it's more like 2x2x2x2. I'm not very mathematical, but I know the difference between addition and multiplication—and the farther you go, the bigger it gets!)

But how do you get a new habit to take root when you've been going the wrong direction for several years? You want a simple answer? Here it is: Two parts to it.

Companionship and accountability.

Actually, they're two sides of the same coin.

Why do you think Weight Watchers has been such a phenomenally successful program for several decades? Companionship and accountability.

Worldwide, Alcoholics Anonymous holds the record for recovering alcoholics. Why do you suppose that is? And from the AA program has come a multitude of other 12 Step programs with similar success rates.

When you're re-programming your subconscious (which is where habits live), you need a lot of repetition and support. The invisible (your unconscious habits) must become very, very visible to you. Every time you're about to _____ (you fill in the blank) scoop out the ice cream, pop a chocolate kiss, guzzle some tap water, bypass the gym and head for the couch, suddenly you become very aware of what you're about to do. A visible habit turns back into—a choice. And that dynamic works best when a group of friends are hanging out together, touching base with each other, and holding each other accountable.

If you're making habit changes on your own, I wish you luck. But you're swimming upstream without a buddy and that's a harder way to go. The statistics aren't on your side. It's much better to make a game of it with a partner, or more than one. Hold each other's feet to the fire. Create a reward when you succeed each week and a price to pay if you don't. One reason it's hard to change a habit is because there's no immediate consequence either way. To win, you've got to set up your own immediate consequences. It feels like a game. But it works.

Here's another tip. Always start out with a commitment you're sure you can keep. Don't do the all-or-nothing thing. That's a recipe for failure. Sometime in your growing up someone probably said to you (usually more than once and with a tone of disgust) that "if you aren't willing to do something right, don't bother doing it at all."

That doesn't work when you're creating new habits. I can't tell you how many positive habits I didn't create because I told myself that I would start when I was ready to "do it right." Big mistake. If you do that, you'll never start. Or if you do, you won't last.

So I've revised my philosophy. Here's my new one: Better to do something positive (even if it's not "right") than not to do it at all. That'll get you started, and you can work up from there.

My friend, Pat, and I set up a game recently where we each committed to 10 minutes of aerobic exercise every single day. If she does hers every day and I don't, I have to buy her dinner the next time we go out. If I do mine and she doesn't, she buys mine. So far, I've bought hers once and she hasn't bought mine at all. I've noticed that when I'm tempted to cop out, the sting of that little consequence gets me off the couch. (Obviously, the long term benefits of exercise don't motivate me nearly as much as not wanting to buy Pat's dinner ever again.)

Companionship is powerful. Companionship with accountability is a lifesaver.

My hope is that one day there will be Wellness Teams springing up that meet together and support each other, just like AA, and Weight Watchers, and the thousands of 12 Step groups do all over this country. I can see hundreds and thousands of enthusiastic Wellness Teams reaching out to one another across telephone lines and internet connections until there are Wellness Communities growing up in every city, state, and nation.

We will be the ones who take the next step into the future and bring health to the rest of the world. We'll be inspired. We'll be educated. And we'll help each other not to forget and not to quit. We will be the leaders of the Wellness Revolution.

Chapter Eight

Affording Wellness

If someone swiped your check register and credit card statements to discover your true priorities, how high up would wellness be?

Eight

Bob and I were driving down the road as he recounted his frustration with his buddy's response to the important new research he'd shared with him.

"He said it made sense. He was impressed with the science behind it. And then he said he couldn't afford it." I wasn't sure if Bob was irritated or sad. "He showed me his new truck and said the payments were eating him up. I don't get it. The doctors say he's got six months to live. How can a new truck be more important than his own body?"

"People have different priorities, Bob." I didn't know what else to say.

We were quiet for a long time. I knew what we both were thinking. If the doctors were right, six months from now his buddy wouldn't even need his truck. Six months later they were right, and he didn't. We don't talk about it much. But we can't help but wonder if it could have been otherwise.

I've heard if you want to see a person's priorities, look at their checkbook. That's where they show up best.

But our priorities aren't necessarily something we consciously choose. Most of them sort of happen on their own. Growing up in our society, we value whatever we're taught to value. We're conditioned to think in a certain way, and our priorities follow suit.

In the health arena, for example, we'll take prescriptions that cost us (and our insurance company) thousands of dollars a year without much more than a shrug and a groan. But whoever heard of budgeting in a Wellness Program? That's not part of our conditioning.

In my own life, I paid more to keep my car running than I was willing to pay to keep my body in good repair. But let's don't talk about my conditioning, that's too embarrassing. Let's talk about yours.

I'm guessing you have a car—how much do you pay to drive that gorgeous vehicle you're going to trade off in a few years? Let's see, there's the initial cost, of course, (in those easy monthly payments if you financed), and then there's registration, inspection, insurance, gasoline, oil, maintenance, tires. Have you ever stopped to add it all up? Not many people do. Why not? Because if you have a car, all that is just part of the deal. And if you neglect any of the above, you know you'll pay a bigger price than if you just take care of it.

But let's say you start treating your car more like you treat your body. Don't give it the fuel it's designed to use—just filled it up with whatever's handy and cheap. And don't bother with the oil and water, either. If the engine light comes on, you can always check into it then. Meanwhile, keep driving. You're too busy to stop and air the tires, or change the belts and spark plugs. Just keep driving till something snaps or goes flat.

Tell me, how healthy will that car be in a few years?

But you wouldn't dream of doing that. Because you've learned to take care of your car. It's part of your conditioning.

But when it comes to taking care of this amazing vehicle that's been your best friend on this earth since you were born; that carries you faithfully every minute of every day—that helps you play with your children and grandchildren, and go to church, and bounce a basketball, and see the sunset, and enjoy a good laugh with your friends—the only vehicle you won't trade in until you're finally ready to check out—well, now, that's another matter. You have to see what you can afford. But you certainly couldn't invest as much as you're paying for your car. After all, you can't live without a car.

Ironic, isn't it? But that's how we think—until something big goes wrong.

My friend had a neighbor who got pancreatic cancer a few years ago. She was 36 years old with 3 young children. The doctors wanted to try a new form of chemotherapy that wasn't yet covered by insurance. The cost was going to be thousands and thousands of dollars. She and her husband would have to take out a second mortgage on their house to pay for it. They did. It didn't save her. But when they took out that second mortgage, it wasn't so much to pay for the chemo as to buy a few more days of hope.

Here's the point: We rarely put an accurate value on (much less invest in) what we take for granted... until we're on the verge of losing it.

Some people call it human nature. I call it conditioning.

But whatever it is, we don't have to let it hypnotize us. We don't have to let it lead us blindly down the primrose path to autoimmune conditions, and cancer, and diabetes, and heart disease.

We are human beings that can wake up. We can educate ourselves. We can stop and re-think. We can change our priorities. And we can take care of our bodies at least as well as we take care of our cars.

Oh yes, one more thing. We can get some help with that. I'm not talking about a government program (thank God) or health insurance either. I've always wondered why they call it health insurance anyway, since it doesn't insure your health and it only pays when you get sick.

There are a hundred companies out there competing for the right to help us afford to be sick—but is there any one out there that will help us afford to be well?

As a matter of fact, there is.

Chapter Nine

Sharing the Gift

Wellness is entirely up to us.
It's a consumer revolution.
We are the army.
We are also the recruiters.

Nine

We like to call it "sharing the gift." Bob shared it with me three years ago now. So what's the gift? It's a paradigm shift. A whole new way of thinking: It is consciously, purposely creating wellness instead of assuming you're healthy until something goes wrong.

Of course, in some cases, something has already gone wrong. Is it too late then? Definitely not. It's never too late to change your programming—to switch your modus operandi from "treating sickness" to "creating wellness."

Treating sickness is what pharmaceuticals are designed to do. They address specific symptoms. They interrupt (or override) the body's natural processes in order to produce a certain result. Most homeopathic remedies do that too. They're not something your body needs all the time in order to do its job. They are temporary "fixes." One of my more knowledgeable friends calls them "bandaids."

Most people assume, if they are handling their symptoms with various remedies, that equates to healthy. My friend, Bob, was taking six different medications to deal with his high blood pressure, arthritis, cholesterol, and I can't remember the rest of them. But if anyone ever asked him (they never did) if he was healthy, he would have said, "Sure." After all, his symptoms were under control, and he wasn't sick, so he considered himself healthy enough.

That's a common assumption. But a good look at the statistics tells a different story. The vast majority of Americans are struggling with symptoms that indicate underlying problems that are neither determined nor addressed. Yet we are treating our symptoms to the tune of $425 billion a year in prescription drugs, according to the most recent data. That's an average of 14 prescriptions per person.

And here's a scary piece of news—the age group with the highest rise in prescriptions issued was—2 to 6 year olds.

Millions of children are fed Ritalin daily in order to deal with symptoms we call ADD and ADHD. And yet the underlying causes remain undetermined. Likewise, with auto-immune diseases. Treatments? We've got 'em. Underlying causes? Sorry, we don't know.

Meanwhile, back at the ranch, the 4th leading cause of death in America turns out to be none other than properly prescribed pharmaceuticals. And 1.5 million people died or were injured from medical treatment. Did you get that? Not a hundred. Not a thousand. Not a hundred thousand. A million and a half.

But again, our conditioning has taught us to accept it. If a million of our soldiers died in battle in a whole decade, much less a single year, the national outcry would be unimaginable. But this? Hey, this is back page news, if you can find it at all.

So, who's going to turn the tide? Who's going to change the direction we're going? It's not the pharmaceutical companies. Frankly, it would be a financial disaster for them if causes were eliminated. Their ongoing profits lie in treating symptoms—starting, preferably, as young as possible and lasting, hopefully, for the rest of your life. Lifetime customers are always the best kind.

Medical institutions certainly aren't going to do it. Nicholas Webb, well known author of "The Cost of Being Sick," became disillusioned with the medical industry when technology he'd developed that allowed diabetics to avert dialysis was rejected because the hospitals needed the money dialysis provided.

Sickness is big business in America.

So, who is going to turn the tide?

We are. We the people. One at a time, we can share the gift with each other—starting, preferably, as early as possible, and lasting, hopefully, the rest of our lives. It's up to us—the consumers—to rise up in our own defense.

And we are not alone. There are companies out there that will help us. Right now they may seem like Davids compared to the Goliaths that rule the Sickness industry. But you know how that story ends, don't you? And as we take up the gauntlet, they will grow stronger too. These companies take Wellness seriously. That's their mission.

They're helping us fight the battle for Wellness in a marketplace addicted to the profits from our sickness. And if we will help them carry the message—and educate the people—they will share their profits with us.

How long has it been since a pharmaceutical company sent you a thank-you check for all the business you've given them over the years? (Are you laughing?) How about your hospital, doctor, surgeon? If you refer your family or friends to their expensive and expert care, you can expect a discount next time, right? Wrong.

Ain't gonna happen.

But the Wellness Revolution is consumer driven. We're the drivers. Just everyday people helping everyday people understand exactly what it takes to be well on purpose. Not well by default. Not assumedly well because you don't feel any symptoms yet. Well on purpose. Consciously. Intentionally.

Because you meant to, you learned how to, and you did it—on purpose.

What if we turned the tables on the Sickness industry by making it not only affordable, but profitable for the consumer to not only get well and stay well themselves—but to help other people do the same? What do you think might happen then?

I'll tell you what might happen.

People might start asking their doctors how to prevent disease instead of waiting to find out what happens once they have it. They might ask them if they've attended a Glycomics Conference to catch up on the now documented information about monosaccharides and cell-to-cell communication. And the doctors who responded by knitting their eyebrows and shaking their heads might just lose some business.

Then, they might start asking around to find the doctors who do know about these things. They might want to talk to medical professionals who have as much interest in causes and prevention as they do in symptoms and treatment.

Sharing the Gift

As consumers, I can see us becoming extremely picky. We'd shop more at stores with organic food aisles. We'd buy meat and eggs from free range animals whenever possible. We'd refuse to drink tap water—even at restaurants. Our favorite eating establishments would serve filtered water without charge.

Whenever we purchased supplements, we'd ask the enlightened questions. Does the manufacturer use GMP's? What function in the body does this have? Is this nutrient (or class of nutrients) absolutely necessary, or merely an enhancement? May I see the research behind it, please? And if the sales person you're talking to stares at you blankly, you know that's not the route to go.

I've been amazed these last three years to find how simple wellness really is. You don't need 25 jars of vitamins in your cupboard. There are actually only a few things your body really needs. But the few things it does need, it NEEDS absolutely. You can't cheat your body and expect it to do its job. Believe me; it will try its hardest. But the ceiling on what it can do to repair and restore, is very often the ceiling you put on it.

Not too long ago I talked with a woman who has years of experience working for a non-profit that helps children struggling with serious illnesses and genetic disorders. The charity provides them with the biologically active monosaccharides (called glyconutrients) that are so necessary for the body to function optimally. I had seen many before-and-after photos that were inspiring and I knew Peggy had seen many miracles.

"Peggy," I said, "I have a friend whose niece has a learning disability that's a little out of the ordinary." I described the problem in as much detail as I could and asked if she thought the glyconutrients they were using could help.

Peggy looked at me and smiled. "If you're asking if they will work—they will. They always work. They do exactly what they're supposed to do. They glycosylate cells so cell-to-cell communication can take place. After that, it's up to the body to determine what happens next. And I can't tell you what that will look like."

If I looked disheartened, it was only for a moment, because she continued. "That's been the most exciting part for us. We've seen the body repair things we never dreamed could be repaired. We've seen genetic conditions reverse that we didn't think could be reversed. The body's ability to create health from almost any condition when it has the right tools has blown our minds over and over again."

"So I can't tell you exactly what will happen. But I can tell you this: The body absolutely needs it. That's all you need to know."

That conversation lives in my mind and speaks to me whenever I hesitate to share nutritional information with someone who's struggling with something. Whenever that old fear crops up and says, "Shhh, you don't need to say anything—how do you know it will help?" Peggy's encouraging words come alive again, because what she said is true—not just about glyconutrients, but about every micronutrient the body needs.

In the last three years I can't even count the number of people I've shared information with who have seen their bodies make wonderful changes.

What is even more wonderful is that they've gone on to share information with others—and they've had the same joy I've had—the joy of watching the miracle of wellness unfold.

And yet it's not really miraculous—at least not in the supernatural sense. It's simply how it was always meant to be. Wellness was a gift God meant for us to have from the beginning. It's our birthright as His kids. We just lost track of it along the way. I think you could say He's trying to get it back to us. But His hands are our hands—and it's our responsibility—and privilege—to share it with each other.

I was speaking with a missionary lady just the other night about glyconutrients, and how crucial they are. Since I know her income is small and unpredictable, I mentioned that if she helped some other folks by sharing information, the thank-you checks would likely cover the cost of what she needed herself. "Well," she said, "I can't really vouch for it until I'm sure it's helping me."

"You don't need to vouch for it," I told her. "The research has already been done. Patents aren't granted without plenty of scientific research and validation. Besides, with a satisfaction guarantee, the bigger risk is not trying it at all. Why not share the information and let them choose for themselves?"

"You're right." she said. "They deserve to know. And they shouldn't have to wait for my results before they do."

Sharing a gift is simple. It's not a sales pitch. There's nothing to "vouch" for – although there are indeed thousands who have already had their lives transformed. It's just a matter of deciding you will not be part of the sick and the tired; that you're ready to start the Wellness journey for yourself—and you're willing to encourage someone else who'd like to do that too.

It begins with believing that it's right—and possible.

It grows stronger with the gathering of knowledge.

It gathers momentum as we reach out to others and share the gift.

The gift is a new way of thinking:

We think we can be healthy.

Wellness Power

We think we can be strong.
And we think it's our responsibility.
Wellness Power.
That's the gift.

Chapter Ten

Stress Free for Real

How much stress would disappear if, no matter what you did from now on, you knew your basic expenses were handled?
That's the power of residual income.

Ten

Everyone knows by now that stress is a health problem. Its very presence acidifies your body, which creates a hazardous environment. Proper pH balance is important (in case you didn't know that) and when you're stressed, it throws you out of balance in that arena.

They've tested it. It's a fact. Traffic, loud noises, harsh words, worry, anxiety, conflict, bad news—they all throw a kink in your pH balance. Your body reacts to all of them by squirting too much acid into that human aquarium that you are. And the fluid environment your cells float around in is a crucial factor in determining how healthy your cells can get. Imagine how some beautiful tropical fish would feel if you squirted acid in their tank every day and didn't clean it out. After while they wouldn't like you very much.

That's how your cells feel when you overdose on acidifying foods (like meat and fried stuff and things that come in boxes)—and then add to it the big S that almost everybody experiences daily. **Stress.** And guess what one of the biggest stressors (other than poor health) is? Finances.

Ah, but you knew that, didn't you? You've probably been there at some point. Maybe you still are. I know I was. Flash back to me a few years ago: Single mom raising two kids. First husband died at 31. Second husband, in the military and too young to be married (at least to be married to me) and left when I was pregnant. Yikes.

You want to talk about financial stress? We can definitely talk.

But something happened that changed my life. Residual income. I now believe everyone should have at least one of those. Talk to some financial planners and see if they don't agree with me on that. Residual income. In case you're not familiar with it, that's money that keeps on coming in from something you already did. It comes in, whether you're working or not. In fact, as it grows larger it gives you a choice whether to work or not.

But even in smaller amounts, residual income is a big stress reliever. Think about it for a minute. What would it feel like to know that your mortgage payment (or your rent or whatever) was handled, permanently. That's one worry you never have to have again.

How would that feel? Stop and think about it. Would that take a bit of the load off your shoulders? Would some of that acidifying stress disappear? It would indeed. I can testify to that.

And you don't have to get rich to be rid of financial stress. You just have to get in a position where your finances don't hinge on your personal effort from now till eternity.

That's why I fell in love with networking years ago. I had already figured out that having a business of your own was the best position to be in as far as taxes were concerned. A CPA friend of mine taught me that.

"Everybody needs to have some sort of personal home-based business," he said. "It's hard for me to watch so many people letting Uncle Sam siphon off so much of their hard-earned money when they should be getting most of it back. Any kind of business would do the trick—it wouldn't matter if they made potholders and sold them on E-Bay. They just need something that's their own."

"So, why don't they?" I asked him.

"They're too busy to think about it," he answered. "I think they're so stressed out with what they're already doing that it's too much trouble to think about anything else. But it costs them a lot. It really does."

No kidding.

And the highest price they pay is the stress itself.

I hate to think where my health or my finances would be today if I hadn't taken my friend's good advice. I'd probably still be fighting traffic to get to my cubicle in some corporate office (that's assuming I made it through all the downsizing and economic cut-backs!) But I haven't had to think about any of that because I did take his advice. And today I'm a huge advocate for home-based business and residual income.

In fact, I'm writing this book because I hope that you'll seriously consider doing two things that will dramatically change the quality of your life for the rest of your life:

1. Take proactive responsibility for your own personal wellness
2. Create a residual income from a home-based business

And if you're so inclined, you can do both at once—just connect with what I believe is one of the most significant grass roots movements going on right now—what economist and author Paul Zane Pilzer calls The Wellness Revolution. That, by the way, is a book worth reading.

My generation—the baby boomers—are grown up now. Only in years, however, not in spirit! And we want to stay as youthful and energetic as we possibly can in the decades ahead. We certainly don't want to wind up in a nursing home if it can be avoided! And our own children—the younger generations coming up behind us—feel exactly the same way.

In the not-so-good-old days, our aging elders just took the health hits as they came without much complaining. Getting old was painful and that's just the way it was. But my generation (and our children) doesn't want to play that game. We're waking up from our stressed-out, fast-food, genetically-modified, nutrient-deficient nightmare. We've given our heads a shake and we're taking the wheel of this miraculous vehicle we live in. We're taking control—and we're doing it now—before we crash and burn.

Something really good is happening in this country—and not only here, but around the world. And it's something we can be part of. The most powerful force in this country is sitting in our chairs. It's who we are—the vast network of every day consumers. We're the people who tell the market exactly what we want by where we spend our dollars. When we spend $500 a month on cars—they build us more cars, fancier cars, better cars. When we spend $4 a day on a cup of coffee, they build another Starbucks.

And when we spend hundreds and even thousands of dollars a year on medications, they give us more drugs.

But guess what will happen when thousands of us start directing our dollars toward high quality products that put our bodies back in balance? You got it. They'll sit up and take notice. When we pass up the grocery store (and even the health food store) vitamin tablets made in chemical laboratories—and instead we opt for actual food-based nutrients—things will change even faster than they are already.

Did you hear that New York City passed a law that demanded the discontinuance of trans-fats in all their restaurants? Hey, that's a big deal. And it didn't happen because the food corporations or the restaurants thought it was a good idea. It happened because the everyday consumers stood up on their hind legs and demanded it.

Let me share something I've discovered from personal experience. If you want to be stress free for real, there are only a few things that are necessary.

First, get real and know that your life is like it is because that's where your choices have allowed it to go. No blaming now (not even of yourself.) Just know it's you behind the wheel of that vehicle. No one else is driving.

Second, take charge. Look at the priorities you're operating with and see if they're the ones you want, or if they're just left over from your conditioning. Reset them if you need to. Make your priorities your own and realign your life along those lines.

Third, get proactive in health and money. Those are the two biggest areas of stress for most of us. Find someone who's been successful in pulling their lives out of the ditch, both health-wise and financially, and ask them to mentor you. (If you could have done it on your own, you already would have.)

Fourth, check out your spiritual connection. If there's no electricity going back and forth in that dimension, you're operating on limited battery power and you'll wear yourself out. It's important to have a live wire in that arena—a spiritual connection that is constantly infusing you with confidence, energy, and good ideas.

Spirituality is a personal, interior thing. It doesn't happen because you go to church (or don't go to church) or because you believe what someone told you once (or twice, or over and over again for 50 years.) You have to develop your own personal understanding—and it's worth the trouble to dig into that. Again, it's a good idea to find someone whose life is clearly full of love and joy and ask them what they know about spiritual things. As always, the way to get good advice is to ask someone who already has the quality of life you're after.

That's about it.

Have I done all those things myself? I have indeed. That's why I'm so confident in sharing these things with you. Because of my home-based business, my tax liability went dramatically south and my income went up. Residual became my favorite word.

When I took charge of my health and started sharing what I'd discovered with a few others, I saw their health take a positive turn. I found out the next best thing to feeling good yourself is watching people you care about start feeling good too. And when I saw them pass on the information to people they cared about, my happiness got even bigger. I began to understand that whatever you give out eventually comes back to you in waves of joy.

I won't say much about the spiritual connection—it's personal. But I will say this: Without that, none of this would have happened like it did. It's just something I know. And every day I thank God for the privilege of experiencing that connection the way I do. It's the light that makes my days sparkle and shine—and the one thing that finally and forever ended my life of stress and left me stress-free for real.

Chapter Eleven

It's Your Call

No one's saying it's a cakewalk.

But if a little lady like Rosa Parks can spark a movement that winds up changing a nation…so can we.
Let's do it.

Eleven

So, how do we boil all this down into a neat little package?

I know some of you are reading this chapter first because you want to get to the bottom line. Hey, you can't get by me, my friend. I'm one of you! And frankly, none of the other chapters matter anyway if you're not willing to get up out of the old armchair and do something you haven't been willing to do before.

Getting up the gumption (my grandmother's phrase) to boldly take charge of your own health and finances is something nobody else can do for you. If you've previously relegated that responsibility to your doctor or your employer, it's time to wake up and smell the coffee.

Neither your doctor nor your employer will be there when you finally run out of health or money, or both. Before that time comes, I'm sure they'll do whatever they can to help you out—as long as it fits within certain parameters. But unless you've taken some bold, specific steps to make sure your body and your bank balance stay fit, one inevitable day you'll find yourself up the proverbial creek with no proverbial paddle.

Personally, I think it's a God-send that there are ways to shore up both our health and finances and get legitimate tax deductions in the process—not to mention generating residual income to boot. But whether you take advantage of that—or whether you don't—it's totally your call.

If all you do is redirect the money you spend on cokes and coffee and cookies and potato chips (and all such nutrient-less sippees and munchies) toward organic foods and nutrient rich supplements, you'll be half-way home. And you can do that. You know you can.

Glyconutrients, phytosterols, anti-oxidants, vitamin/minerals, and Omega 3's are absolutely necessary for your body to function properly. That's just all there is to it. And pro-biotics and enzymes help your digestive tract absorb them. Just make sure you get them from a reputable source that's quality controlled by GMP's and third party tested for standardization. Most health food store brands are not.

The important thing to know is this: It's your call. But it's more than just you that hangs in the balance. It's your family, your children and grandchildren, your friends and their families, the next generation—frankly, I'm not sure where the ripple ends.

But I believe that, together, we can make a change in the direction we're going.

If one of us (like me, for instance, and whoever gave you this book) will encourage a few good friends to grab hold of the wheel of their own life because they really matter to us and we want them to live long and joyfully—then the dominos can start falling to the positive side—and the Wellness Revolution can gain momentum, one friend at a time.

Let's face it. Our society has built a huge financial infrastructure around a consumer population that has traded our good health for a bag of cheetos and a cola. If we all took hold of the wheel of our lives and actually reclaimed our own well being, some of those structures would begin to topple. And multi-billion dollar industries are not interested in seeing their own demise.

That's why what we're up to isn't quite a cake-walk.

The opposition is entrenched and financially well-armed. No, they'll never come right out and state that their monetary ideal is a chronically sick society that only functions with the help of ongoing pharmaceutical remedies. But anyone who can read a profit and loss statement and understands the goal of business doesn't need any help to see that.

Nevertheless, money and power have never had the final word when it comes to what's right and wrong. In the end, the power always lies in the hands of the people themselves. It's our call.

Just think, if a little lady like Rosa Parks can spark a fire that winds up righting a wrong that was deeply entrenched for hundreds of years—what can a few of us who care about bringing health back to the world do if we decide to?

Rosa refused to give up her seat. I refuse to give up my health.

What about you?

Epilogue

Never doubt that a small group of thoughtful, committed citizens can change the world. Indeed, it is the only thing that ever has.
> —*Margaret Mead*

You must be the change you want to see in the world.
> —*Mahatma Gandhi*

>> Yes, we can.
>> It's worth it.
>> And it's time.

Suggested Reading

Sugars That Heal: The New Healing Science of Glyconutrients by Emil Mondoa

Live Better, Longer: The Science Behind the Amazing Healh Benefits of OPC by Richard Passwater

Drug-Induced Nutrient Depletion Handbook by Ross Pelton and James LaValle

Prescription for Nutritional Healing: A Practical A-to-Z Reference to Drug-Free Remedies

What Your Doctor Doesn't Know About Nutritional Medicine May Be Killing You by Ray Strand

The Healing Power of 8 Sugars: An Amazing Breakthrough in Nutrition, Sciences and Medicine by Allan C. Somersall

The Pycnogenol Phenomenon: The Most Unique & Versatile Health Supplement by Peter Rohdewald

The Omega-3 Effect: Everything You Need to Know About the Super Nutrient for Living Longer, Happier, and Healthier by William Sears

Enzymes for Autism and Other Neurological Conditions (Updated Third Edition) by Karen DeFelice

The Truth About Statins: Risks and Alternatives to Cholesterol-Lowering Drugs by Barbara Roberts

Vitamin C: The Real Story – The Remarkable and Controversial Healing Factor by Steve Hickey

Miracle Sugars: The Glyconutrient Link to Disease Prevention and Improved Health by Rita Elkins

The Mind-Gut Connection: How the Hidden Conversation Within Our Bodies Impacts Our Mood, Our Choices, and Our Overall Health by Emeran Mayer

The Wellness Revolution by Paul Zane Pilzer

Made in the USA
Middletown, DE
12 July 2019